Mediterranean Cooking Guide

Wholesome and Mouth-Watering Recipes
for a perfect and Healthy lifestyle

Lara Dillard

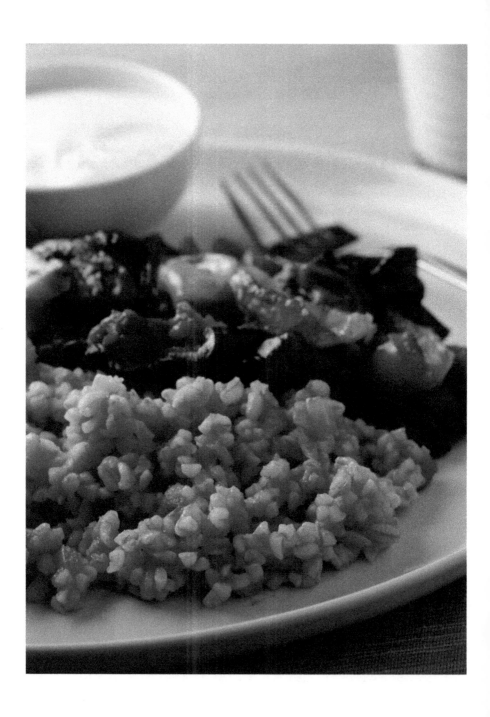

by reading this document, the reader agrees that under no circumstances is the author responsible for any losses, direct or indirect, which are incurred as a result of the use of information contained within this document, including, but not limited to, — errors, omissions, or inaccuracies.

Table of Contents

Greek Ginger-Blackberry Bulgur

Difficulty Level: 1/5

Preparation time: *10 minutes*

Cooking time: *0 minutes*

Servings: *4*

Ingredients:

¼ cup bulgur

¼ tsp. ground ginger

⅔ plain low-fat yogurt

2 tbsp honey

3 tbsp refrigerated coconut milk

¼ cup blackberries

Directions:

Combine and stir together the first five ingredients in a mixing bowl. Divide mixture evenly between two ½-pint jars. Top it with blackberries.

Cover the jars and refrigerate them overnight, or up to

a maximum of 3 days. Stir before serving.

Nutrition:

Calories: 215

Total Fats: 1g

Fiber: 3g

Carbohydrates: 45g

Protein: 8g

Energizing Eggs with Tomato Toppings & Spinach Sauté

Difficulty Level: 2/5

Preparation time: **25 minutes**

Cooking time: **5 minutes**

Servings: **4**

Ingredients:

12-pcs egg whites

½-cup skim milk

½-tsp salt

¼-tsp ground black pepper

1-tbsp olive oil

1-clove garlic, minced

2-cups fresh baby spinach

2-cups cherry tomatoes, cut in half

¼-cup Parmesan cheese, finely shredded

Directions:

Combine and whisk together the egg whites, skim milk, salt, and pepper in a mixing bowl. Mix until fully combined. Set aside.

Heat the oil in a large nonstick skillet placed over medium-high heat. Add in the garlic; cook and stir for 30 seconds. Add in the spinach and tomatoes; cook and stir about a minute until the tomatoes soften and spinach leaves wilt. Remove from the skillet and keep the mixture warm.

In the same skillet, placed over medium heat, pour the egg white mixture. Cook until the mixture sets without stirring. By using a spatula, lift and fold so that the uncooked portions of the egg mixture flow underneath. Continue cooking for 3 minutes until the egg mixture cooks through but still moist and glossy.

Remove from the heat. To serve, arrange the egg and spinach mixtures on a serving plate. Sprinkle over with cheese.

Nutrition:

Calories: 142

Total Fats: 3g

Fiber: 2g

Carbohydrates: 7g

Protein: 15g

Tabbouleh Tidbits Combo Classic

Difficulty Level: 1/5

Preparation time: **20 minutes**

Cooking time: **0 minutes**

Servings: **6**

Ingredients:

For the Salad:

½-cup whole-wheat bulgur

4-Roma tomatoes, finely chopped and drained of excess juice

4-pcs green onions, very finely chopped

2-bunches parsley, stems removed, washed and well-dried, finely chopped

1-pc English cucumber, finely chopped

12-pcs fresh mint leaves, stems removed, washed, well-dried, finely chopped

Salt

Whole-wheat pita bread (optional)

Romaine lettuce leaves, to serve (optional)

For the Dressing:

3-tbsp lemon juice

3-tbsp extra-virgin olive oil

Directions:

For the Salad:

Rinse the bulgur and soak in water for 7 minutes. Drain thoroughly by squeezing the bulgur to rid excess water. Set aside.

Combine the remainder of the salad ingredients in a large mixing bowl. Mix until fully combined. Add the bulgur and season with salt. Mix again.

For the Dressing:

Combine and whisk together all the dressing ingredients in a mixing bowl. Mix well until fully combined.

Drizzle the dressing over the salad. Toss gently to coat evenly.

Cover and refrigerate the salad for 30 minutes before serving. If desired, serve the tabbouleh salad with a side dish of whole-wheat pita bread and Romaine lettuce leaves, which serve as 'boats' or wraps for the salad.

Nutrition:

Calories: 190

Total Fats: 10g

Fiber: 3.1g

Carbohydrates: 25.5g

Protein: 3.2g

Power Pods & Hearty Hazelnuts with Mustard-y Mix

Difficulty Level: 2/5

Preparation time: *15 minutes*

Cooking time: *15 minutes*

Servings: *4*

Ingredients:

1-lb. green beans, trimmed

3-tbsp extra-virgin olive oil (divided)

2-tsp whole grain mustard

1-tbsp red wine vinegar

¼-tsp salt

¼-tsp ground pepper

¼-cup toasted hazelnuts, chopped

Directions:

Preheat your grill to high heat.

In a large mixing bowl, toss the green beans with a tablespoon of olive oil. Place the beans in a grill basket. Grill for 8 minutes until charring a few spots, stirring occasionally.

Combine and whisk together the remaining oil, mustard, vinegar, salt, and pepper in the same mixing bowl. Add the grilled beans and toss to coat evenly.

To serve, top the side dish with hazelnuts.

Nutrition:

Calories: 181

Total Fats: 15g

Fiber: 9g

Carbohydrates: 9g

Protein: 3g

Chicken Rolls

Difficulty Level: 2/5

Preparation time: 10 minutes

Cooking time: 12 minutes

Servings: 4

Ingredients:

4 chicken breast halves, skinless and boneless

Salt and black pepper to taste

4 teaspoons olive oil

1 small cucumber, sliced

3 teaspoons cilantro, chopped

4 Greek whole wheat tortillas

4 tablespoons peanut sauce

Directions:

Heat a grill pan over medium high heat, season chicken with salt and pepper, rub with the oil, add to the grill, cook for 6 minutes on each side, transfer to a cutting board, cool down and slice.

In a bowl, mix cilantro with cucumber and stir.

Spread 1 tablespoon peanut sauce on each tortilla, divide chicken and cucumber mix on each, fold, arrange on plates and serve.

Nutrition:

Calories: 321,

Fat: 3,

Fiber: 4,

Carbohydrates: 7,

Protein: 9

Cheesy Chicken

Difficulty Level: 2/5

Preparation time: 10 minutes

Cooking time: 15 minutes

Servings: 6

Ingredients:

¼ cup breadcrumbs

¼ teaspoon garlic powder

½ cup pecorino cheese, grated

1 teaspoon basil, dried

3 tablespoons olive oil

A pinch of salt and black pepper

6 chicken breast halves, skinless and boneless

Directions:

In a bowl, mix breadcrumbs with garlic powder, cheese, basil, salt and pepper and stir.

Rub chicken with half of the oil and dip in breadcrumbs..

Heat a pan with remaining oil over medium high heat, add the meat, cook for 7 minutes, flip, cook for 8 minutes more, divide between plates and serve, with a side salad.

Nutrition:

Calories: 212,

Fat: 2,

Fiber: 1,

Carbohydrates: 3,

Protein: 18

Chicken and Onion and Mustard Sauce

Difficulty Level: 2/5

Preparation time: 10 minutes

Cooking time: 20 minutes

Servings: 4

Ingredients:

8 bacon strips, cooked and chopped

1/3 cup mustard

1 cup yellow onion, chopped

1 tablespoon olive oil

1 and ½ cups chicken stock

4 chicken breasts, skinless and boneless

¼ teaspoon sweet paprika

Directions:

In a bowl, mix the chicken with paprika with mustard, salt and pepper and stir well.

Heat the a pan with the oil over medium high heat, add chicken breasts, cook for 2 minutes on each side and also transfer to a plate.

Heat the pan once again over medium high heat, add stock, bacon, onions, salt and pepper, stir and bring to a simmer.

Return chicken to pan as well, stir gently and simmer over medium heat for 20 minutes, turning meat halfway.

Divide chicken on plates, drizzle the sauce over it and serve.

Nutrition:

Calories: 223,

Fat: 8,

Fiber: 1,

Carbohydrates: 3,

Protein: 26

Chicken and Peppers Mix

Difficulty Level: 2/5

Preparation time: 10 minutes

Cooking time: 20 minutes

Servings: 4

Ingredients:

4 teaspoons pine nuts, toasted

1 pound chicken breasts, skinless, boneless

2 tablespoons white flour

Cooking spray

¼ cup shallots, chopped

¼ cup roasted peppers, chopped

2 tablespoons capers, chopped

2 tablespoons black olives, pitted and sliced

1 cup orange juice

1 tablespoon lemon juice

1 cup chicken stock

A pinch of salt and black pepper

2 tablespoons parsley, chopped

Directions:

Pound chicken breasts into ½-inch thick pieces, add salt and pepper, dredge them in flour. Heat a pan over medium-high heat and grease with cooking spray.

Add the chicken, cook for 2 minutes on each side and transfer to a plate.

Heat up the same pan over medium heat, add the shallots and the rest of the ingredients except the parsley, stir and sauté for 5 minutes.

Return the chicken to the pan, cook everything for 8 minutes more, divide between plates, sprinkle the parsley on top and serve.

Nutrition:

Calories: 223,

Fat: 10,

Fiber: 5,

Carbohydrates: 15,

Protein: 8

Chicken and Pineapple Platter

Difficulty Level: 2/5

Preparation time: 10 minutes

Cooking time: 10 minutes

Servings: 4

Ingredients:

20 ounces canned pineapple slices

A drizzle of olive oil

3 cups chicken thighs, boneless, skinless and cut into medium pieces

1 tablespoon smoked paprika

Directions:

Heat a pan over medium high heat, add pineapple slices, cook them for a few minutes on each side, transfer to a cutting board, cool them down and cut into medium cubes.

Heat another pan with a drizzle of oil over medium high heat, rub chicken pieces with paprika, add them to the pan, cook for 5 minutes on each side, arrange it on a platter, top with the pineapple and serve.

Nutrition:

Calories: 120,

Fat: 3,

Fiber: 1,

Carbohydrates: 5,

Protein: 2

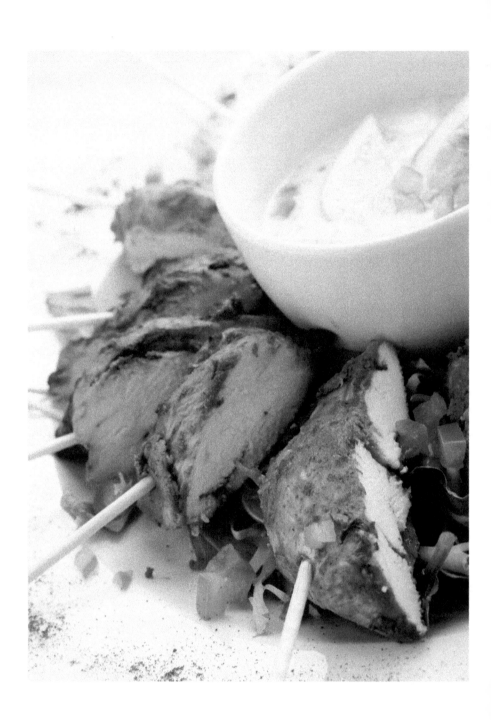

Chicken, Apple and Cucumber Sandwich

Difficulty Level: 1/5

Preparation time: 10 minutes

Cooking time: 0 minutes

Servings: 6

 Ingredients:

½ cup hot water

1 celery stalk, chopped

½ cup mayonnaise

1 red apple, cored and chopped

½ cup smoked chicken breast, skinless, boneless, cooked and shredded

1 teaspoon thyme, chopped

1 cucumber, sliced

12 whole grain bread slices, toasted

Sunflower sprouts

Directions:

In a bowl, mix chicken with celery and the other ingredients except the bread and the sprouts and stir well.

Divide this into 6 bread slices, add sunflower sprouts on each, top with the other bread slices and serve.

Nutrition:

Calories: 160,

Fat: 7,

Fiber: 2,

Carbohydrates: 10,

Protein: 5

Creamy Chicken and Tomato Mix

Difficulty Level: 1/5

Preparation time: 10 minutes

Cooking time: 20 minutes

Servings: 4

Ingredients:

5 chicken thighs

1 tablespoon olive oil

1 tablespoon thyme, chopped

2 garlic cloves, minced

1 teaspoon red pepper flakes, crushed

½ cup heavy cream

¾ cup chicken stock

½ cup sun dried tomatoes in olive oil, drained and chopped

Salt and black pepper to taste

¼ cup parmesan cheese, grated

Basil leaves, chopped for serving

Directions:

Heat a pan with the oil over medium high heat, add chicken, salt and pepper to taste, cook for 3 minutes on each side, transfer to a plate and leave aside for now.

Return pan to heat, add thyme, garlic and pepper flakes, stir and cook for 1 minute.

Add the rest of the ingredients except the basil, stir and bring to a simmer.

Add chicken pieces, stir, place in the oven at 350 degrees F and bake for 15 minutes.

Divide between plates and serve with basil sprinkled on top.

Nutrition:

Calories: 212,

Fat: 4,

Fiber: 3,

Carbohydrates: 3,

Protein: 3

Creamy Chicken and Grapes

Difficulty Level: 1/5

Preparation time: 10 minutes

Cooking time: 0 minutes

Servings: 6

Ingredients:

20 ounces chicken meat, already cooked and chopped

½ cup pecans, chopped

1 cup green grapes, seedless and cut in halves

½ cup celery, chopped

ounces canned mandarin oranges, drained

For the creamy cucumber salad dressing:

1 cup Greek yogurt

1 cucumber, chopped

1 garlic clove, chopped

Salt and white pepper to taste

1 teaspoon lemon juice

Directions:

In a bowl, mix cucumber with the chicken, salt, pepper to taste, lemon juice and the other ingredients, toss and keep in the fridge until you serve it.

Nutrition:

Calories: 200,

Fat: 3,

Fiber: 1,

Carbohydrates: 2,

Protein 8

Chicken with Cheese and Cabbage Mix

Difficulty Level: 2/5

Preparation time: 10 minutes

Cooking time: 6 minutes

Servings: 4

Ingredients:

3 medium chicken breasts, skinless, boneless and cut into thin strips

4 ounces green cabbage, shredded

5 tablespoon extra virgin olive oil

Salt and black pepper to taste

2 tablespoons sherry vinegar

1 tablespoon chives, chopped

¼ cup feta cheese, crumbled

¼ cup barbeque sauce

2 bacon slices, cooked and crumbled

Directions:

In a bowl, mix the cabbage with 4 tablespoon oil with vinegar, salt and pepper to taste and stir well.

Season chicken with salt and pepper, heat a pan with remaining oil over medium high heat, add chicken, cook for 6 minutes, take off heat, transfer to a bowl, add barbeque sauce and toss.

Arrange between plates, add chicken strips, sprinkle cheese, chives and bacon and serve.

Nutrition:

Calories: 200,

Fat: 15,

Fiber: 3,

Carbohydrates: 10,

Protein: 33

Parmesan Chicken and Zucchini Mix

Difficulty Level: 2/5

Preparation time: 10 minutes

Cooking time: 15 minutes

Servings: 4

Ingredients:

1 pound chicken breasts, cut into medium chunks

12 ounces zucchini, sliced

2 tablespoons olive oil

2 garlic cloves, minced

2 tablespoons parmesan, grated

1 tablespoon parsley, chopped

Salt and black pepper to taste

Directions:

In a bowl, mix chicken pieces with 1 tablespoon oil, some salt and pepper and toss to coat.

Heat a pan over medium high heat, add chicken pieces, brown for 6 minutes on all sides, transfer to a plate and leave aside.

Heat the pan with the remaining oil over medium heat, add zucchini slices, garlic, return the chicken, sprinkle the parmesan on top, stir and cook for 5 minutes.

Divide between plates and serve with some parsley on top.

Nutrition:

Calories: 212,

Fat: 4,

Fiber: 3,

Carbs: 4,

Protein 7

Lime Chicken and Corn Salad

Difficulty Level: 2/5

Preparation time: 10 minutes

Cooking time: 20 minutes

Servings: 2

 Ingredients:

2 tablespoons olive oil

2 ounces quinoa

2 ounces cherry tomatoes, cut in quarters

3 ounces sweet corn

A handful coriander, chopped

Lime juice from 1 lime

Lime zest from 1 lime, grated

Salt and black pepper to taste

2 spring onions, chopped

1 small red chili pepper, chopped

1 avocado, pitted, peeled and chopped

7 ounces chicken meat, roasted, skinless, boneless and chopped

Directions:

Put some water in a pan, bring to a boil over medium high heat, add quinoa, stir and cook for 12 minutes.

Meanwhile, put corn in a pan, heat over medium high heat, cook for 5 minutes and leave aside for now.

Drain quinoa, transfer to a bowl, add the meat and the rest of the ingredients, toss and serve.

Nutrition:

Calories: 320,

Fat: 4,

Fiber: 4,

Carbohydrates: 5,

Protein: 7

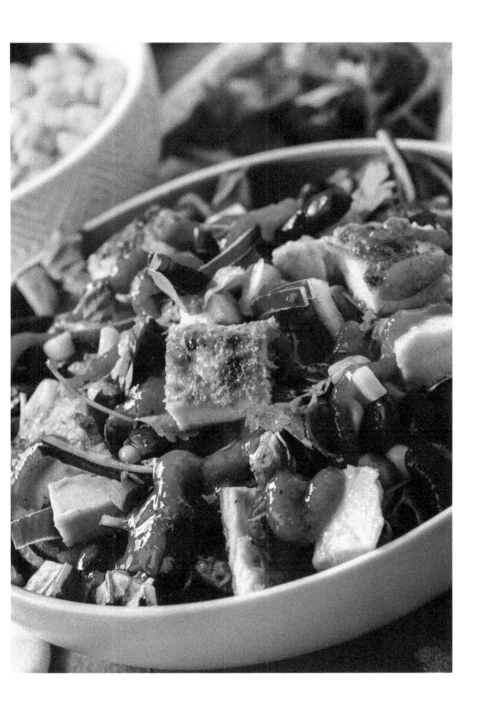

Lemon Lentils

Difficulty Level: 2/5

Preparation time: 10 minutes

Cooking time: 20 minutes

Servings: 6

 Ingredients:

1 cup brown lentils

1 cup carrots, chopped

1 cup red onions, chopped

2 tablespoons lemon juice

½ cup celery, cubed

¼ cup parsley, chopped

2 garlic cloves, minced

A pinch of salt and black pepper

½ teaspoon thyme, dried

¼ cup olive oil

Directions:

Place the lentils in a pot, add carrots, onions, celery, salt, pepper, thyme, cover with water, bring to a boil and simmer over medium heat for 20 minutes.

Drain well, put the mix into a bowl, add garlic, parsley, salt, pepper and the oil, toss and serve.

Nutrition:

Calories: 170,

Fat: 7,

Fiber: 3,

Carbohydrates: 12,

Protein: 6

Cabbage and Carrots Salad

Difficulty Level: 1/5

Preparation time: 10 minutes

Cooking time: 0 minutes

Servings: 4

Ingredients:

1 green cabbage head, shredded

A pinch of salt and black pepper

3 carrots, shredded

1 yellow bell pepper, chopped

1 orange bell pepper, chopped

1 red bell pepper, chopped

8 kalamata olives, pitted and chopped

2 tablespoons white vinegar

2 tablespoons olive oil

Directions:

In a bowl, mix the cabbage with salt, pepper and the other ingredients, toss and serve.

Nutrition:

Calories: 150,

Fat: 9,

Fiber: 4,

Carbohydrates; 8,

Protein: 8

Pomegranate Salad

Difficulty Level: 1/5

Preparation time: 10 minutes

Cooking time: 0 minutes

Servings: 3

Ingredients:

3 big pears, cored and cut with a spiralizer

¾ cup pomegranate seeds

5 ounces arugula

¾ cup walnuts, chopped

For the vinaigrette:

1 tablespoon sesame oil

1 tablespoon olive oil

1 tablespoon maple syrup

1 teaspoon white sesame seeds

2 tablespoons apple cider vinegar

1 tablespoon soy sauce

1 garlic clove, minced

A pinch of sea salt

Black pepper to taste

Directions:

In a bowl, mix the pears with the pomegranate seeds, arugula and all the other ingredients, toss to coat well and serve right away.

Nutrition:

Calories: 200,

Fat: 2,

Fiber: 4,

Carbohydrates: 6,

Protein: 9

Maple Chickpeas Mix

Difficulty Level: 1/5

Preparation time: 15 minutes

Cooking time: 0 minutes

Servings: 2

Ingredients:

16 ounces canned chickpeas, drained

1 handful raisins

1 handful baby spinach leaves

1 tablespoon maple syrup

½ tablespoon lemon juice

4 tablespoons olive oil

1 teaspoon cumin, ground

A pinch of sea salt

Black pepper to taste

½ teaspoon chili flakes

Directions:

In a bowl, mix maple syrup with lemon juice, oil, cumin, a pinch of salt, black pepper and chili flakes and whisk well.

In a salad bowl, mix chickpeas with spinach, the rest of the ingredients and the salad dressing, toss and serve.

Nutrition:

Calories: 300,

Fat: 3,

Fiber: 6,

Carbohydrates: 12,

Protein: 9

Berry and Yogurt Parfait

Difficulty Level: 1/5

Preparation time: 5 minutes

Cooking time: 0 minutes

Servings: 2

Ingredients:

1 cup raspberries

1½ cups unsweetened nonfat plain Greek yogurt

1 cup blackberries

¼ cup chopped walnuts

Directions:

In 2 bowls, layer the raspberries, yogurt, and blackberries. Sprinkle with the walnuts.

Nutrition:

Calories: 290;

Protein: 29g;

Total Carbohydrates: 27g;

Sugars: 12g;

Fiber: 10g;

Total Fat: 10g;

Saturated Fat: <1g;

Cholesterol: 15mg;

Sodium: 92mg

Yogurt with Blueberries, Honey, and Mint

Difficulty Level: 1/5

Preparation time: 5 minutes

Cooking time: 0 minutes

Servings: 2

Ingredients:

2 cups unsweetened nonfat plain Greek yogurt

1 cup blueberries

3 tablespoons honey

2 tablespoons fresh mint leaves, chopped

Directions:

Apportion the yogurt between 2 small bowls. Top with the blueberries, honey, and mint.

Nutrition:

Calories: 314;

Protein: 15g;

Total Carbohydrates: 54g;

Sugars: 50g; Fiber: 2g;

Total Fat: 3g;

Saturated Fat: 3g;

Cholesterol: 15mg;

Sodium: 175mg

Almond and Maple Quick Grits

Difficulty Level: 2/5

Preparation time: 5 minutes

Cooking time: 6 minutes

Servings: 4

Ingredients:

1½ cups water

½ cup unsweetened almond milk

Pinch sea salt

½ cup quick-cooking grits

½ teaspoon ground cinnamon

¼ cup pure maple syrup

¼ cup slivered almonds

Directions:

In a medium saucepan over medium-high heat, heat the water, almond milk, and sea salt until it boils.

Stirring constantly with a wooden spoon, slowly add the grits. Continue stirring to prevent lumps and bring the mixture to a slow boil. Reduce the heat to medium-low.

Simmer for 5 to 6 minutes, stirring frequently, until the water is completely absorbed.

Stir in the cinnamon, syrup, and almonds. Cook for 1 minute more, stirring.

Nutrition:

Calories: 151;

Protein: 3g;

Total Carbohydrates: 28g;

Sugars: 12g;

Fiber: 3g;

Total Fat: 4g;

Saturated Fat: <1g;

Cholesterol: 0mg;

Sodium: 83mg

Oatmeal with Berries and Sunflower Seeds

Difficulty Level: 2/5

 Preparation time: 5 minutes

Cooking time: 10 minutes

Servings: 4

Ingredients:

1¾ cups water

½ cup unsweetened almond milk

Pinch sea salt

1 cup old-fashioned oats

½ cup blueberries

½ cup raspberries

¼ cup sunflower seeds

Directions:

In a medium saucepan over medium-high heat, heat the water, almond milk, and sea salt to a boil.

Stir in the oats. Reduce the heat to medium-low and

cook, stirring occasionally, for 5 minutes. Cover, and let the oatmeal stand for 2 minutes more. Stir and serve topped with the blueberries, raspberries, and sunflower seeds.

Nutrition:

Calories: 186;

Protein: 6g;

Total Carbohydrates: 32g;

Sugars: 4g;

Fiber: 5g;

Total Fat: 4g;

Saturated Fat: <1g;

Cholesterol: 0mg;

Sodium: 96mg

French Toast

Difficulty Level: 2/5

Preparation time: 20 minutes

Cooking time: 10 minutes

Servings: 6

Ingredients:

1½ cups unsweetened almond milk

2 eggs, beaten

2 egg whites, beaten

1 teaspoon vanilla extract

Zest of 1 orange

Juice of 1 orange

1 teaspoon ground nutmeg

6 light whole-wheat bread slices

Nonstick cooking spray

Directions:

In a small bowl, whisk the almond milk, eggs, egg whites, vanilla, orange zest and juice, and nutmeg.

Arrange the bread in a single layer in a 9-by-13-inch baking dish. Pour the milk and egg mixture over the top. Allow the bread to soak for about 10 minutes, turning once.

Spray a nonstick skillet with cooking spray and heat over medium-high heat. Working in batches, add the bread and cook for about 5 minutes per side until the custard sets.

Nutrition:

Per Serving (1 slice)

Calories: 223;

Protein: 8g;

Total Carbohydrates: 15g;

Sugars: 6g;

Fiber: 5g;

Total Fat: 21g;

Saturated Fat: 13g;

Cholesterol: 55mg;

Sodium: 126mg

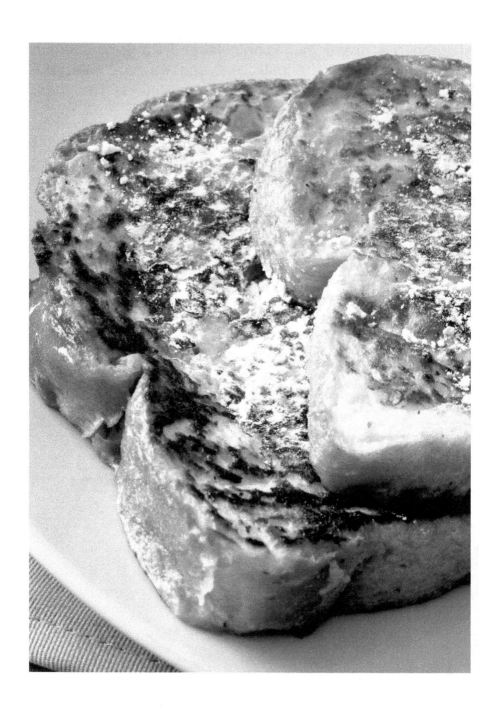

Tomato and Zucchini Frittata

Difficulty Level: 2/5

Preparation time: 10 minutes

Cooking time: 18 minutes

Servings: 4

Ingredients:

3 eggs

3 egg whites

½ cup unsweetened almond milk

½ teaspoon sea salt

⅛ teaspoon freshly ground black pepper

2 tablespoons extra-virgin olive oil

1 zucchini, chopped

8 cherry tomatoes, halved

¼ cup (about 2 ounces) grated Parmesan cheese

Directions:

Heat the oven's broiler to high, adjusting the oven rack to the center position.

In a small bowl, whisk the eggs, egg whites, almond milk, sea salt, and pepper. Set aside.

In a 12-inch ovenproof skillet over medium-high heat, heat the olive oil until it shimmers.

Add the zucchini and tomatoes and cook for 5 minutes, stirring occasionally.

Pour the egg mixture over the vegetables and cook for about 4 minutes without stirring until the eggs set around the edges.

Using a silicone spatula, pull the set eggs away from the edges of the pan. Tilt the pan in all directions to allow the unset eggs to fill the spaces along the edges. Continue to cook for about 4 minutes more without stirring until the edges set again.

Sprinkle the eggs with the Parmesan. Transfer the pan to the broiler. Cook for 3 to 5 minutes until the cheese melts and the eggs are puffy. Cut into wedges to serve.

Nutrition:
Calories: 223;

Protein: 14g;

Total Carbohydrates: 13g;

Sugars: 8g;

Fiber: 4g;

Total Fat: 4g;

Saturated Fat: 4g;

Cholesterol: 133mg;

Sodium: 476mg

Smoked Salmon Scramble

Difficulty Level: 2/5

Preparation time: 5 minutes

Cooking time: 10 minutes

Servings: 4

Ingredients:

4 eggs

6 egg whites

⅛ teaspoon freshly ground black pepper

2 tablespoons extra-virgin olive oil

½ red onion, finely chopped

4 ounces smoked salmon, flaked

2 tablespoons capers, drained

Directions:

In a small bowl, whisk the eggs, egg whites, and pepper. Set aside.

In a large nonstick skillet over medium-high heat, heat the olive oil until it shimmers.

Add the red onion and cook for about 3 minutes, stirring occasionally, until soft.

Add the salmon and capers and cook for 1 minute.

Add the egg mixture to the pan and cook for 3 to 5 minutes, stirring frequently, or until the eggs are set.

Nutrition:

Calories: 189;

Protein: 16g;

Total Carbohydrates: 2g;

Sugars: 1g;

Fiber: <1g;

Total Fat: 13g;

Saturated Fat: 2g;

Cholesterol: 170mg;

Sodium: 806mg

Poached Eggs with Avocado Purée

Difficulty Level: 2/5

Preparation time: 10 minutes

Cooking time: 5 minutes

Servings: 4

Ingredients:

2 avocados, peeled and pitted

¼ cup chopped fresh basil leaves

3 tablespoons red wine vinegar, divided

Juice of 1 lemon

Zest of 1 lemon

1 garlic clove, minced

1 teaspoon sea salt, divided

⅛ teaspoon freshly ground black pepper

Pinch cayenne pepper, plus more as needed

4 eggs

Directions:

In a blender, combine the avocados, basil, 2 tablespoons of vinegar, the lemon juice and zest, garlic, ½ teaspoon of sea salt, pepper, and cayenne. Purée for about 1 minute until smooth.

Fill a 12-inch nonstick skillet about three-fourths full of water and place it over medium heat. Add the remaining tablespoon of vinegar and the remaining ½ teaspoon of sea salt. Bring the water to a simmer.

Carefully crack the eggs into custard cups. Holding the cups just barely above the water, carefully slip the eggs into the simmering water, one at a time. Turn off the heat and cover the skillet. Let the eggs sit for 5 minutes without agitating the pan or removing the lid.

Using a slotted spoon, carefully lift the eggs from the water, allowing them to drain completely. Place each egg on a plate and spoon the avocado purée over the top.

Nutrition:
Calories: 213;

Protein: 2g;

Total Carbohydrates: 11g;

Sugars: <1g;

Fiber: 7g;

Total Fat: 20g;

Saturated Fat: 4g;

Cholesterol: 0mg;

Sodium: 475mg

Sweet Potato Mash

Difficulty Level: 2/5

Preparation time: 10 minutes

Cooking time: 20 minutes

Servings: 6

Ingredients:

4 sweet potatoes, peeled and cubed

¼ cup almond milk

¼ cup extra-virgin olive oil

½ teaspoon sea salt

⅛ teaspoon freshly ground black pepper

Directions:

In a large pot over high heat, combine the sweet potatoes with enough water to cover by 2 inches. Bring the water to a boil. Reduce the heat to medium and cover the pot. Cook for 15 to 20 minutes until the potatoes are soft.

Drain the potatoes and return them to the dry pot off the heat. Add the almond milk, olive oil, sea salt, and pepper. With a potato masher, mash until smooth.

Nutrition:
 Calories: 243;

Protein: 2g;

Total Carbohydrates: 35g;

Sugars: 5g;

Fiber: 5g;

Total Fat: 11g;

Saturated Fat: 3g;

Cholesterol: 0mg;

Sodium: 169mg

No-Mayo Florence Tuna Salad

Difficulty Level: 1/5

Servings: 4

Preparation Time: **10 minutes**

Ingredients:

4 cups spring mix greens

1 (15-ounce) can cannellini beans, drained

2 (5-ounce) cans water-packed, white albacore tuna, drained (I prefer Wild Planet brand)

⅔ cup crumbled feta cheese

½ cup thinly sliced sun-dried tomatoes

¼ cup sliced pitted kalamata olives

¼ cup thinly sliced scallions, both green and white parts

3 tablespoons extra-virgin olive oil

½ teaspoon dried cilantro

2 or 3 leaves thinly chopped fresh sweet basil

1 lime, zested and juiced

Kosher salt

Freshly ground black pepper

DIRECTIONS:

In a large bowl, combine greens, beans, tuna, feta, tomatoes, olives, scallions, olive oil, cilantro, basil, and lime juice and zest. Season with salt and pepper, mix, and enjoy!

VARIATION TIP: What I love about this dish is that the swap-ins are endless. Is the family getting bored with cannellini beans? Try replacing 50 percent of the beans with lentils or chickpeas. Baby kale or spinach instead of arugula is a great way to introduce different phytonutrients into your diet while adding some variety to this lunch at the same time.

Nutrition:

Per serving (1 cup)

Calories: 355

Protein: 22g

Total Carbohydrates: 25g

Sugars: 5g

Fiber: 8g

Total Fat: 19g

Saturated Fat: 5g

Cholesterol: 47mg

Sodium: 744mg

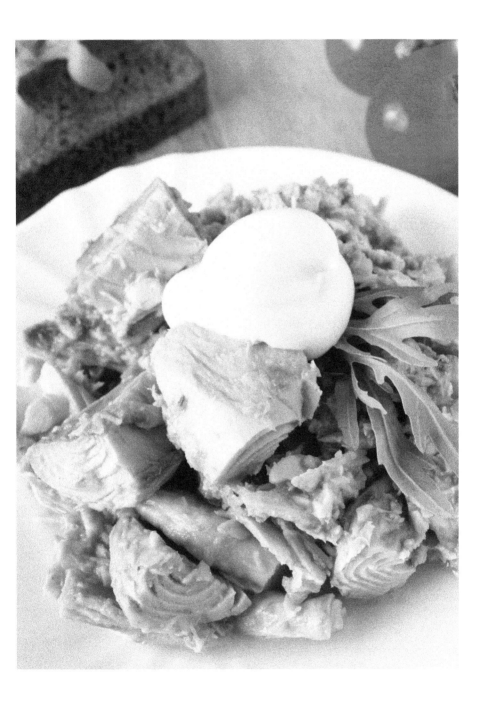

Shakshuka Bake

Difficulty Level: 2/5

Servings: 4

Preparation time: **5 minutes**

Cooking time: **20 minutes**

Ingredients:

2 tablespoons extra-virgin olive oil

1 cup chopped shallots

1 cup chopped red bell peppers

1 cup finely diced potato

1 teaspoon garlic powder

1 (14.5-ounce) can diced tomatoes, drained

¼ teaspoon turmeric

¼ teaspoon paprika

¼ teaspoon ground cardamom

4 large eggs

¼ cup chopped fresh cilantro

Directions:

Preheat the oven to 350°F.

In an oven-safe sauté pan or skillet, heat the olive oil over medium-high heat and sauté the shallots, stirring occasionally, for about 3 minutes, until fragrant. Add the bell peppers, potato, and garlic powder. Cook, uncovered, for 10 minutes, stirring every 2 minutes.

Add the tomatoes, turmeric, paprika, and cardamom to the skillet and mix well. Once bubbly, remove from heat and crack the eggs into the skillet so the yolks are facing up.

Put the skillet in the oven and cook for an additional 5 to 10 minutes, until eggs are cooked to your preference. Garnish with the cilantro and serve.

VARIATION TIP: For a spicy shakshuka, add ¼ teaspoon red pepper flakes while heating up the diced tomatoes.

Nutrition:

Per serving

Calories: 224

Protein: 9g

Total Carbohydrates: 20g

Sugars: 7g

Fiber: 3g

Total Fat: 12g

Saturated Fat: 3g

Cholesterol: 186mg

Sodium: 278mg

Morning Glory Muffins

Difficulty Level: 2/5

Servings: 12

Preparation time: **5 minutes**

Cooking time: **15 minutes**

Ingredients:

Nonstick cooking spray

1½ cups granulated sugar

½ cup brown sugar

¾ cup all-purpose flour

2 teaspoons pumpkin pie spice

1 teaspoon baking soda

¼ teaspoon salt

Pinch nutmeg

3 mashed bananas

1 (15-ounce) can pure pumpkin puree

½ cup plain, unsweetened, full-fat yogurt

½ cup (1 stick) butter, melted

2 large egg whites

Directions:

Preheat the oven to 350°F. Spray a muffin tin with cooking spray.

In a large bowl, mix the sugars, flour, pumpkin pie spice, baking soda, salt, and nutmeg. In a separate bowl, mix the bananas, pumpkin puree, yogurt, and butter. Slowly mix the wet ingredients into the dry ingredients.

In a large glass bowl, using a mixer on high, whip the egg whites until stiff and fold them into the batter.

Pour the batter into a muffin tin, filling each cup halfway. Bake for 15 minutes, or until a fork inserted in the center comes out clean.

LEFTOVER TIP: These make a great weekday breakfast on the go. Store them in individual bags for portion control, or toast and butter one if you have the 5 minutes to spare. They last 3 to 5 days in an airtight container.

Nutrition:

Per serving

Calories: 259

Protein: 3g

Total Carbohydrates: 49g

Sugars: 36g

Fiber: 3g

Total Fat: 8g

Saturated Fat: 5g

Cholesterol: 22mg

Sodium: 226mg

C+C French Toast

Difficulty Level: 2/5

Servings: 6

Preparation time: **5 minutes**

Cooking time: **15 minutes**

Ingredients:

1 cup whole milk

3 large eggs

2 teaspoons grated orange zest

1 teaspoon vanilla extract

⅛ teaspoon ground cardamom

⅛ teaspoon ground cinnamon

1 loaf of boule bread, sliced 1 inch thick (gluten-free preferred)

1 banana, sliced

¼ *cup* Berry and Honey Compote

Directions:

Heat a large nonstick sauté pan or skillet over medium-high heat.

In a large, shallow dish, mix the milk, eggs, orange zest, vanilla, cardamom, and cinnamon. Working in batches, dredge the bread slices in the egg mixture and put in the hot pan.

Cook for 5 minutes on each side, until golden brown. Serve, topped with banana and drizzled with honey compote.

LEFTOVER TIP: Reheat the French toast, covered with a damp paper towel, in the microwave oven the next day in 10-second increments.

Nutrition:

Per serving

Calories: 414

Protein: 17g

Total Carbohydrates: 78g

Sugars: 15g

Fiber: 3g

Total Fat: 6g

Saturated Fat: 2g

Cholesterol: 98mg

Sodium: 716mg

South of the Coast Sweet Potato Toast

Difficulty Level: 2/5

Servings: 4

Preparation time: **5 minutes**

Cooking time: **15 minutes**

Ingredients:

2 plum tomatoes, halved

6 tablespoons extra-virgin olive oil, divided

Salt

Freshly ground black pepper

2 large sweet potatoes, sliced lengthwise

1 cup fresh spinach

8 medium asparagus, trimmed

4 large cooked eggs or egg substitute (poached, scrambled, or fried)

1 cup arugula

4 tablespoons pesto

4 tablespoons shredded Asiago cheese

Directions:

Preheat the oven to 450°F.

On a baking sheet, brush the plum tomato halves with 2 tablespoons of olive oil and season with salt and pepper. Roast the tomatoes in the oven for approximately 15 minutes, then remove from the oven and allow to rest.

Put the sweet potato slices on a separate baking sheet and brush about 2 tablespoons of oil on each side and season with salt and pepper. Bake the sweet potato slices for about 15 minutes, flipping once after 5 to 7 minutes, until just tender. Remove from the oven and set aside.

In a sauté pan or skillet, heat the remaining 2 tablespoons of olive oil over medium heat and sauté the fresh spinach until just wilted. Remove from the pan and rest on a paper-towel-lined dish. In the same pan, add the asparagus and sauté, turning throughout. Transfer to a paper towel-lined dish.

Place the slices of grilled sweet potato on serving plates and divide the spinach and asparagus evenly among the slices. Place a prepared egg on top of the spinach and asparagus. Top this with ¼ cup of arugula.

Finish by drizzling with 1 tablespoon of pesto and sprinkle with 1 tablespoon of cheese. Serve with 1 roasted plum tomato.

PREPARATION TIP: Prep the ingredients (except eggs) the day before and make this delicious dish in a flash in the morning. Just reheat the ingredients in the oven, add your eggs, top, and enjoy.

Nutrition:

Per serving

Calories: 441

Protein: 13g

Total Carbohydrates: 23g

Sugars: 9g

Fiber: 4g

Total Fat: 35g

Saturated Fat: 7g

Cholesterol: 217mg

Sodium: 481mg

Falafel Bites

Difficulty Level: 2/5

Servings: 4

Preparation time: **15 minutes**

Cooking time: **15 minutes**

Ingredients:

1⅔ cups falafel mix

1¼ cups water

Extra-virgin olive oil spray

1 tablespoon pickled onions (optional)

1 tablespoon pickled turnips (optional)

2 tablespoons Tzatziki sauce (optional)

Directions:

In a large bowl, carefully stir the falafel mix into the water. Mix well. Let stand 15 minutes to absorb the water. Form mix into 1-inch balls and arrange on a baking sheet.

Preheat the broiler to high.

Take the balls and flatten slightly with your thumb (so they won't roll around on the baking sheet). Spray with olive oil, and then broil for 2 to 3 minutes on each side, until crispy and brown.

To fry the falafel, fill a pot with ½ inch of cooking oil and heat over medium-high heat to 375°F. Fry the balls for about 3 minutes, until brown and crisp. Drain on paper towels and serve with pickled onions, pickled turnips, and Tzatziki sauce (if using).

INGREDIENT TIP: It's really important to let the mix rest until the liquid is absorbed or else you won't be able to make patties that hold together.

Nutrition:

Per Serving

Calories: 166

Protein: 17g

Total Carbohydrates: 30g

Sugars: 5g

Fiber: 8g

Total Fat: 2g

Saturated Fat: 0g

Cholesterol: 0mg

Sodium: 930mg

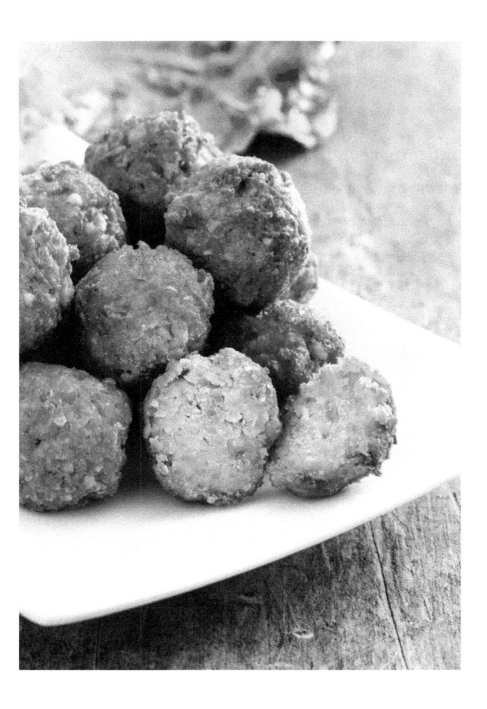

Spring Mix with Fig and Citrus Dressing

Difficulty Level: 1/5

Servings: 2

Preparation time: **10 minutes**

Ingredients:

¼ cup Skinny Cider Dressing

4 cups spring mix greens

⅓ cup crumbled goat cheese

3 tablespoons fig jam

2 to 3 heirloom tomatoes, cut into 3-inch chunks

1 to 2 tablespoons balsamic glaze

6 slices prosciutto, rolled

Directions:

In a large bowl, drizzle the dressing over the salad greens, and toss well.

In a separate bowl, whisk the goat cheese and jam together and set aside.

Put the salad mix in serving bowls, top with the tomatoes, then drizzle the cheese mixture over dish.

Finish the dish with a drizzle of balsamic glaze and top with the prosciutto.

INGREDIENT TIP: If you regularly refrigerate your balsamic glaze, make sure it returns to room temperature before using it in a salad.

Nutrition:

Per serving

Calories: 375

Protein: 23g

Total Carbohydrates: 30g

Sugars: 24g

Fiber: 3g

Total Fat: 15g

Saturated Fat: 7g

Cholesterol: 77mg

Sodium: 2,160mg

Tricolor Tomato Summer Salad

Difficulty Level: 1/5

Servings: 3-4

Preparation time: **10 minutes**

Ingredients:

¼ cup while balsamic vinegar

2 tablespoons Dijon mustard

1 tablespoon sugar

½ teaspoon freshly ground black pepper

½ teaspoon garlic salt

¼ cup extra-virgin olive oil

1½ cups chopped orange, yellow, and red tomatoes

½ cucumber, peeled and diced

1 small red onion, thinly sliced

¼ cup crumbled feta (optional)

Directions:

In a small bowl, whisk the vinegar, mustard, sugar, pepper, and garlic salt. Next, slowly whisk in the olive oil.

In a large bowl, add the tomatoes, cucumber, and red onion. Add the dressing. Toss once or twice, and serve with feta crumbles (if using) on top.

PREP TIP: If you want to prep this recipe ahead of time, store the dressing separately from the salad until you are ready to serve it.

Nutrition:

Per serving

Calories:

Protein: 246g

Total Carbohydrates: 19g

Sugars: 13g

Fiber: 2g

Total Fat: 18g

Saturated Fat: 3g

Cholesterol: 0mg

Sodium: 483mg

Almond Flour Pancakes with Berry and Honey Compote

Difficulty Level: 2/5

Preparation time: **5 minutes**

Cooking time: **15 minutes**

Servings: 4

Ingredients:

1 cup almond flour

1 cup plus 2 tablespoons skim milk

2 large eggs, beaten

⅓ cup honey

1 teaspoon baking soda

¼ teaspoon salt

2 tablespoons extra-virgin olive oil

1 sliced banana or 1 cup sliced strawberries, divided

2 tablespoons Berry and Honey Compote

Directions:

In a bowl, mix together the almond flour, milk, eggs, honey, baking soda, and salt.

In a large sauté pan or skillet, heat the olive oil over medium-high heat and pour ⅓ cup pancake batter into the pan. Cook for 2 to 3 minutes. Right before pancake is ready to flip, add half of the fresh fruit and flip to cook for 2 to 3 minutes on the other side, until cooked through.

Top with the remaining fruit, drizzle with Berry and Honey Compote and serve.

Nutrition:

Per serving

Calories: 415

Protein: 12g

Total Carbohydrates: 46g

Sugars: 38g

Fiber: 4g

Total Fat: 24g

Saturated Fat: 3g

Cholesterol: 94mg

Sodium: 526mg

Spanish Potato Salad

Difficulty Level: 2/5

Preparation time: 10 minutes

Cooking time: 10 minutes

Servings: 6 to 8

Ingredients:

4 russet potatoes, peeled and chopped

3 large hard-boiled eggs, chopped

1 cup frozen mixed vegetables, thawed

½ cup plain, unsweetened, full-fat Greek yogurt

5 tablespoons pitted Spanish olives

½ teaspoon freshly ground black pepper

½ teaspoon dried mustard seed

½ tablespoon freshly squeezed lemon juice

½ teaspoon dried dill

Salt

Freshly ground black pepper

Directions:

Boil potatoes for 5 to 7 minutes, until just fork-tender, checking periodically for doneness. You don't want to overcook them.

While the potatoes are cooking, in a large bowl, mix the eggs, vegetables, yogurt, olives, pepper, mustard, lemon juice, and dill. Season with salt and pepper. Once the potatoes are cooled somewhat, add them to the large bowl, then mix well and serve.

LEFTOVER TIP: This dish tastes even better the next day, after the flavors have time to set overnight. It makes for a great meal prepping recipe.

Nutrition:

Per serving

Calories: 192

Protein: 9g

Total Carbohydrates: 30g

Sugars: 3g

Fiber: 2g

Total Fat: 5g

Saturated Fat: 1g

Cholesterol: 96mg

Sodium: 59mg

Curry Zucchini Soup

Difficulty Level: 2/5

Preparation time: **10 minutes**

Cook time: **20 minutes**

Servings: 4 to 6

Ingredients:

¼ cup extra-virgin olive oil

1 medium onion, chopped (about ½ cup)

1 carrot, shredded

1 small garlic clove, minced

4 cups low-sodium chicken broth

2 medium zucchini, thinly sliced

2 apples, peeled and chopped

2½ teaspoons curry powder

¼ teaspoon salt

Directions:

In a large pot, heat the oil over medium heat. Sauté the onion, carrot, and garlic and cook until tender. Add the chicken broth, zucchini, apples, and curry powder.

Boil for 2 minutes, reduce the heat, and simmer for 20 minutes, until the vegetables are tender.

Season with the salt and serve.

INGREDIENT TIP: You can prep the carrots, garlic, onion, and zucchini up to 3 days in advance to reduce prep time on the day of cooking.

LEFTOVER TIP: You can freeze this soup for up to 6 months.

Nutrition:

Per serving

Calories: 208

Protein: 4g

Total Carbohydrates: 19g

Sugars: 11g

Fiber: 4g

Total Fat: 14g

Saturated Fat: 2g

Cholesterol: 0mg;

Sodium: 237mg

Rustic Winter Salad

Difficulty Level: 1/5

Preparation time: **10 minutes**

Servings: 4

Ingredients:

1 small green apple, thinly sliced

6 stalks kale, stems removed and greens roughly chopped

½ cup crumbled feta cheese

½ cup dried currants

½ cup chopped pitted kalamata olives

½ cup thinly sliced radicchio

2 scallions, both green and white parts, thinly sliced

¼ cup peeled, julienned carrots

2 celery stalks, thinly sliced

¼ cup Sweet Red Wine Vinaigrette

Salt (optional)

Freshly ground black pepper (optional)

Directions:

In a large bowl, combine the apple, kale, feta, currants, olives, radicchio, scallions, carrots, and celery and mix well. Drizzle with the vinaigrette. Season with salt and pepper (if using), then serve.

LEFTOVER TIP: Store salad and dressing separately.

VARIATION TIP: Add some grilled chicken and you have a great work lunch. Store the dressing on the side and toss right before eating.

Nutrition:

Per serving

Calories: 253

Protein: 6g

Total Carbohydrates: 29g

Sugars: 19g

Fiber: 4g

Total Fat: 15g

Saturated Fat: 4g

Cholesterol: 17mg

Sodium: 480mg

Yellow and White Hearts of Palm Salad

Difficulty Level: 1/5

Preparation time: **10 minutes**

Servings: 4

Ingredients:

2 (14-ounce) cans hearts of palm, drained and cut into ½-inch-thick slices

1 avocado, cut into ½-inch pieces

1 cup halved yellow cherry tomatoes

½ small shallot, thinly sliced

¼ cup coarsely chopped flat-leaf parsley

2 tablespoons low-fat mayonnaise

2 tablespoons extra-virgin olive oil

¼ teaspoon salt

⅛ teaspoon freshly ground black pepper

Directions:

In a large bowl, toss the hearts of palm, avocado, tomatoes, shallot, and parsley.

In a small bowl, whisk the mayonnaise, olive oil, salt, and pepper, then mix into the large bowl.

INGREDIENT TIP: Add fresh-squeezed lemon juice to brighten up the dish before eating.

Nutrition:

Per serving

Calories: 192

Protein: 5g

Total Carbohydrates: 14g

Sugars: 2g

Fiber: 7g

Total Fat: 15g

Saturated Fat: 2g

Cholesterol: 0mg

Sodium: 841mg

Herby tomato soup

Difficulty Level: 2/5

Preparation time: **10 minutes**

Cooking time: **10 minutes**

Servings: 2

Ingredients:

¼ cup extra-virgin olive oil

2 garlic cloves, minced

1 (14.5-ounce) can plum tomatoes, whole or diced

1 cup vegetable broth

¼ cup chopped fresh basil

Directions:

In a medium pot, heat the oil over medium heat, then add the garlic and cook for 2 minutes, until fragrant.

Meanwhile, in a bowl using an immersion blender or in a blender, puree the tomatoes and their juices.

Add the pureed tomatoes and broth to the pot and mix well. Simmer for 10 to 15 minutes and serve, garnished with basil.

INGREDIENT TIP: If you don't have fresh basil, you can sprinkle dried basil into the soup before serving.

Nutrition:

Per serving

Calories: 307

Protein: 3g

Total Carbohydrates: 11g

Sugars: 10g

Fiber: 4g

Total Fat: 27g

Saturated Fat: 4g

Cholesterol: 0mg

Sodium: 661mg

Cod and Cabbage

Difficulty Level: 2/5

Preparation time: *10 minutes*

Cooking time: **15 minutes**

Servings: *4*

Ingredients:

Cups green cabbage, shredded

Sweet onion, sliced

A pinch of salt and black pepper

½ cup feta cheese, crumbled

Teaspoons olive oil

4 cod fillets, boneless

¼ cup green olives, pitted and chopped

Directions:

Grease a roasting pan with the oil, add the fish, the cabbage and the rest of the *INGREDIENTS*, introduce in the pan and cook at 450 degrees F for 15 minutes.

Divide the mix between plates and serve.

Nutrition:

Calories: 270

Fat: 10g

Fiber: 3g

Carbohydrates: 12g

Protein: 31mg

Baked Chicken

Difficulty Level: 2/5

Preparation time: *5 minutes*

Cooking time: 25 minutes

Servings: *4*

Ingredients:

1 and ½ pounds chicken thighs, boneless and skinless

2 tablespoons harissa paste

½ cup Greek yogurt

Salt and black pepper to taste

1 tablespoon lemon juice

1 tablespoon mint, finely chopped

Directions:

Put chicken thighs in a lined baking dish, add salt and pepper to taste and leave aside for now.

Meanwhile, in a bowl, mix lemon juice with yogurt, salt and pepper and stir.

Add harissa, stir again and spread over chicken pieces. Place chicken thighs in the oven at 165 degrees F and bake for 20 minutes.

Transfer dish to your preheated broiler and broil for 5 minutes.

Divide chicken on plates, sprinkle mint on top and serve.

Nutrition:

Calories: 250

Fat: 12g

Fiber: 0

Carbohydrates: 2g

Protein: 31g

Grilled Chicken and Vinaigrette

Difficulty Level: 2/5

***Preparation time:* 10 minutes**

Cooking time: 10 minutes

Servings: *4*

Ingredients:

2 tablespoon vegetable oil

4 chicken breast halves, skinless and boneless

Salt and black pepper to taste

1 tablespoon shallot, chopped

1 tablespoon vinegar

½ teaspoon sugar

½ teaspoon mustard

6 tablespoons olive oil

2 tablespoons parsley chopped

2 tablespoons kalamata olives, pitted and chopped

Directions:

Place each chicken piece between 2 parchment paper pieces, brush meat with the vegetable oil, season with salt and pepper, place on preheated grill pan, cook for 10 minutes turning once.

Transfer to a cutting board and leave aside for a few minutes.

In a bowl, mix shallot with vinegar, mustard, sugar, salt, pepper, olive oil, parsley and olives and whisk well.

Cut chicken in thin slices, arrange on a platter and serve with the vinaigrette on top.

Nutrition:
Calories: 400

Fat: 32g

 Fiber: 0g

Carbohydrates: 2g

Protein 24g

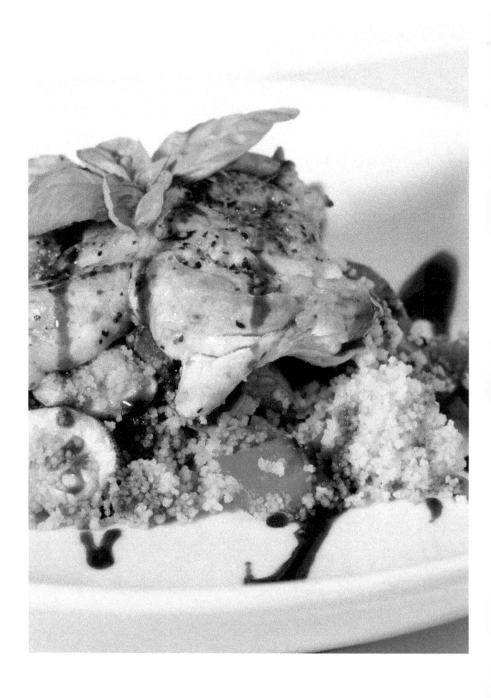